The Complete Slow Cooker Delicacies

Don't Miss These Quick and Easy meat for everyday meals

Donna Conway

© copyright 2021 – all rights reserved.

the content contained within this book may not be reproduced, duplicated or transmitted without direct written permission from the author or the publisher.

under no circumstances will any blame or legal responsibility be held against the publisher, or author, for any damages, reparation, or monetary loss due to the information contained within this book. either directly or indirectly.

legal notice:

this book is copyright protected. this book is only for personal use. you cannot amend, distribute, sell, use, quote or paraphrase any part, or the content within this book, without the consent of the author or publisher.

disclaimer notice:

please note the information contained within this document is for educational and entertainment purposes only. all effort has been executed to present accurate, up to date, and reliable, complete information. no warranties of any kind are declared or implied. readers acknowledge that the author is not engaging in the rendering of legal, financial, medical or professional advice. the content within this book has been derived from various sources. please consult a licensed professional before attempting any techniques outlined in this book.

by reading this document, the reader agrees that under no circumstances is the author responsible for any losses, direct or indirect, which are incurred as a result of the use of information contained within this document, including, but not limited to, — errors, omissions, or inaccuracies.

Table of Contents

Honey Chicken Drumsticks 6

Rosemary Lemon Chicken 8

Rotisserie Chicken 10

Salsa Chicken 12

Turmeric Chicken 13

Marinara Chicken 15

Chocolate Chicken 17

Coconut Curried Chicken 19

Buffalo Chicken 21

Teriyaki Chicken 23

Pulled BBQ Chicken 25

Lemon Thyme Chicken 27

Chicken and Gravy 29

Cilantro Lime Chicken 30

Garlic Chicken 31

Caribbean Jerk Chicken 33

Balsamic Chicken 35

Caesar Chicken 37

Cheesy Cheddar Chicken 39

Lemon Butter Chicken 40

Tahini Chicken 41

Shredded Mexican Chicken 43

Parmesan Chicken Drumsticks 45

Mediterranean Chicken 47

Lemon Garlic Chicken 49

Sweet & Smoky Pulled Chicken 51

Mexican Chicken Fajita Soup 53

CREAMY TUSCAN GARLIC CHICKEN	55
CHICKEN STEW	57
CURRIED CHICKEN TACOS	59
RANCH CHICKEN	62
CHICKEN AND SAUSAGE	64
CRACK CHICKEN	66
CHEESY ADOBO CHICKEN	68
GREEN BEANS & CHICKEN THIGHS	70
PIZZA CHICKEN	72
CHICKEN WITH BACON GRAVY	74
CHICKEN LO MEIN	76
CHICKEN BACON CHOWDER	79
SESAME GINGER CHICKEN	82
COCO LOCO CHICKEN CURRY	84
RANCH CHICKEN WITH BROCCOLI	86
GARLIC PARMESAN CHICKEN WINGS	88
LUAU CHICKEN	90
SOUTHWEST CHICKEN	92
CAROLINA-STYLE VINEGAR CHICKEN	94
CHICKEN CACCIATORE WITH ZOODLES	96
BOK CHOY CHICKEN	98
CHICKEN TIKKA MASALA	100
CHILI LIME CHICKEN WINGS	102
GARLIC CHICKEN & MUSHROOM CHOWDER	104
SAUCY DUCK	107

Honey Chicken Drumsticks

Preparation time: 15 minutes

Cooking time: 6 hours

Servings: 2-4 people

Ingredients:

- 8 chicken drumsticks
- 1 tablespoon honey
- 3 apples, peeled and diced
- ½ teaspoon cinnamon
- 1 teaspoon salt
- Garnish: chopped parsley, sesame seeds

Directions:

1. Rinse the chicken, pat dry. Mix the honey and salt in a medium bowl. Pour mixture over the drumsticks.

2. Place the drumsticks in the slow cooker. Cover and cook on low within 6 hours, until chicken is tender. Serve hot. Garnish with parsley and sesame seeds.

Nutrition:

Calories: 259

Fat: 5.6g

Carbs: 27.7g

Protein: 25.8g

Rosemary Lemon Chicken

Preparation time: 15 minutes

Cooking time: 6 hours

Servings: 4 people

Ingredients:

- 4 pounds of chicken thighs, bone & skin in
- 1 tablespoon olive oil
- Pinch of sea salt and ground black pepper, each
- ½ cup of preferred flour
- 3 medium yellow onions, sliced
- 8 carrots, sliced
- 6 garlic cloves, chopped
- 3 springs rosemary
- ½ cup lime juice
- ¾ cup chicken broth
- 1 tablespoon lemon zest
- 1 lemon sliced

Directions:

1. Rinse the chicken, pat dry. Place the chicken, salt, pepper, onions, carrots in your slow cooker. Sprinkle the flour over ingredients. Stir until they are coated.
2. Add garlic, rosemary, lime juice, broth, lemon zest, sliced lemon. Cover and cook on low within 6 hours, until chicken is tender. Serve hot.

Nutrition:

Calories: 510

Fat: 14g

Carbs: 24.7g

Protein: 63g

Rotisserie Chicken

Preparation time: 15 minutes

Cooking time: 6 hours

Servings: 4 people

Ingredients:

- 5-pound fresh chicken
- 2 tablespoons olive oil
- 4-5 sweet potatoes, small size
- a couple pinches sea salt, fresh ground pepper, each

Directions:

1. Rinse the chicken, pat dry. Coat the chicken with oil. Season with salt and pepper. Coat the potatoes with oil, salt, plus pepper. Wrap in foil.

2. Place the potatoes along the bottom of the slow cooker. Place chicken over the potatoes. Cover and cook on low within 6 hours. Serve hot.

Nutrition:

Calories: 443

Fat: 15.3g

Carbs: 17.4g

Protein: 55.6g

Salsa Chicken

Preparation time: 15 minutes

Cooking time: 6 hours

Servings: 4 people

Ingredients:

- 4 chicken thighs
- salad greens
- 1 pint of salsa
- shredded cheese

Directions:

1. Rinse the chicken, pat dry. Place the chicken, greens, and salsa in the slow cooker. Cook on low for 6 hours. Garnish with cheese.

Nutrition: Calories: 310 Fat: 10.9g Carbs: 7.1g Protein: 44.6g

Turmeric Chicken

Preparation time: 15 minutes

Cooking time: 5 hours

Servings: 4 people

Ingredients:

- 5 pounds of chicken, organic
- 1 teaspoon turmeric
- ½ cup coconut milk, full fat
- 4 garlic cloves, finely grated
- 2-3-inch fresh ginger, grated
- Pinch of salt and fresh ground pepper, each
- Garnish: Scallions

Directions:

1. In the slow cooker, combine the turmeric, ginger, and garlic. Stir in the coconut milk. Season chicken with

salt and pepper. Place in the slow cooker. Cook on low within 5 hours, until chicken cooked. Shred with 2 forks.

Nutrition:

Calories: 359

Fat: 7.7g

Carbs: 2.1g

Protein: 66g

Marinara Chicken

Preparation time: 15 minutes

Cooking time: 4 hours

Servings: 4 people

Ingredients:

- 4 pounds of chicken
- 1 jar marinara sauce
- 1 onion, diced
- 2 garlic cloves, diced
- ½ green pepper, diced
- 2 zucchinis, diced
- ¼ cup basil
- Pinch of salt and fresh ground pepper, each
- Garnish: Parmigiano Reggiano, grated

Directions:

1. Rinse the chicken, pat dry. Season the chicken with salt and pepper. Place in the slow cooker. Add the onions, garlic, green pepper, and zucchini.

2. Pour the marinara sauce over the ingredients. Cover and cook on medium within 4 hours, until cooked through.
3. Shred the chicken with 2 forks. Serve warm over favorite pasta. Top with Parmigiano Reggiano.

Nutrition:

Calories: 319

Fat: 6.1g

Carbs: 8.9g

Protein: 54.5g

Chocolate Chicken

Preparation time: 15 minutes

Cooking time: 6 hours

Servings: 2-4 people

Ingredients:

- 2 pounds chicken breasts, bone-in
- Pinch of sea salt, fresh ground pepper, each
- 2 tablespoons ghee
- 1 medium onion, diced
- 4 garlic cloves, minced
- 7 medium tomatoes, peeled and chopped
- 2 1/2 oz. of dark chocolate, crumbled
- 5 dried chili peppers, finely chopped
- 1 teaspoon cumin powder
- ¼ cup Almond Butter
- ½ teaspoon cinnamon powder
- 1/2 teaspoon guajillo chili powder

- Garnish: diced Avocado, chopped cilantro, and diced jalapeno pepper, seeds out

Directions:

1. Rinse the chicken, pat dry. Place all the other fixings in the slow cooker. Cover and cook on low within 6 hours. Serve warm. Garnish with avocado chunks, cilantro, and diced jalapeno.

Nutrition:

Calories: 477

Fat: 20.6g

Carbs: 19.6g

Protein: 53.4g

Coconut Curried Chicken

Preparation time: 15 minutes

Cooking time: 5 hours

Servings: 4 people

Ingredients:

- 3 pounds of chicken breasts/thighs
- 1 large onion, chopped
- 2 small carrots, chopped
- 2 garlic cloves, minced
- 1 tablespoon curry powder
- 1 tablespoon mustard condiment
- ½ cup coconut cream
- ½ cup chicken stock
- 2 tablespoons ghee
- Pinch of salt
- 2 Yukon gold potatoes, peeled, chopped
- Garnish: chopped parsley

Directions:

1. Rinse the chicken, pat dry. Place all the fixings, except the potatoes, in the slow cooker. Stir well. After 3 hours of cooking, add the potatoes. Cover and cook on low within 4-5 hours, until chicken and potatoes are tender. Serve warm.

Nutrition:

Calories: 377

Fat: 25g

Carbs: 6.3g

Protein: 30.4g

Buffalo Chicken

Preparation time: 15 minutes

Cooking time: 6 hours

Servings: 2-4 people

Ingredients:

- ½ pound chicken breast, boneless, skinless
- ½ pound chicken thighs, boneless, skinless
- 1/3 cup hot sauce
- 1 tablespoon coconut aminos
- 2 tablespoons ghee
- ¼ teaspoon cayenne
- ½ teaspoon garlic powder
- 4 small sweet potatoes, chopped
- ¼ - ½ cup of water
- Garnish: ranch dressing, chives

Directions:

1. Rinse the chicken, pat dry. In a skillet, combine the ghee, garlic powder, hot sauce, cayenne, and coconut aminos. Simmer for 5 minutes.
2. Coat the chicken with the mixture—place in the slow cooker. Add the potatoes, then pour in ¼ cup of water.
3. Cover and cook on low within 5-6 hours, until chicken cooked. Serve warm. Garnish with ranch dressing, chives.

Nutrition:

Calories: 423

Fat: 11.4g

Carbs: 56.4g

Protein: 24.1g

Teriyaki Chicken

Preparation time: 15 minutes

Cooking time: 6 hours

Servings: 4 people

Ingredients:

- 2 pounds chicken thighs, boneless, skinless
- 3 tablespoons honey
- ½ cup coconut aminos
- 1 ½ teaspoons minced ginger
- 4 garlic cloves, minced
- 1 tablespoon sesame seeds, toasted
- 1 teaspoon of sea salt

Directions:

1. Rinse the chicken, pat dry. Place all the fixings, except sesame seeds, in the slow cooker. Cook on low within 5-6 hours, until chicken cooked through.

2. Cut the chicken into bite-size pieces. Garnish with sesame seeds. Serve warm on a bed of rice.

Nutrition:

Calories: 341

Fat: 12g

Carbs: 11.7g

Protein: 44.2g

Pulled BBQ Chicken

Preparation time: 15 minutes

Cooking time: 4 hours

Servings: 2-4 people

Ingredients:

- 3 pounds of chicken breasts
- 2 cups tomatoes, diced
- 3-4 pitted dates
- 3 garlic cloves, minced
- ½ large yellow onion, diced
- 3 tablespoons apple cider vinegar
- 2 teaspoons sea salt
- 1 tablespoon smoked paprika
- 6 oz. tomato paste
- 1 ½ tablespoon avocado oil

Directions:

1. Rinse the chicken, pat dry. Drizzle the chicken with avocado oil. Place in the slow cooker. Blend the rest of the ingredients in a food processor. Pour over chicken. Cook on low for 4 hours. Shred with 2 forks. Serve hot.

Nutrition:

Calories: 217

Fat: 6.3g

Carbs: 19.6g

Protein: 22.1g

Lemon Thyme Chicken

Preparation time: 15 minutes

Cooking time: 4 hours

Servings: 4 people

Ingredients:

- 4-pound chicken
- ¼ cup lemon juice
- 1 teaspoon dried thyme
- 2-3 bay leaves
- 5 garlic cloves, diced
- 1 teaspoon of sea salt
- ¼ teaspoon black pepper
- ¼ cup of water

Directions:

1. Rinse the chicken, pat dry. Place in the slow cooker. Pour lemon juice over the chicken. Season with thyme, salt, and pepper. Add bay leaves, garlic.

2. Put the water in the bottom of the slow cooker. Cover and cook for 4 hours, until chicken is cooked through. Serve hot.

Nutrition:

Calories: 276

Fat: 5.6g

Carbs: 0.3g

Protein: 52.7g

Chicken and Gravy

Preparation time: 10 minutes

Cooking time: 8 hours

Servings: 4 people

Ingredients:

- 2 lbs. chicken breasts, skinless, boneless, and cut into pieces
- 3 cups chicken stock
- 1 oz brown gravy mix
- 1 oz onion soup mix

Directions:

1. Add chicken stock, brown gravy mix, and onion soup mix into the slow cooker and stir well. Add chicken into the slow cooker. Cover and cook on low within 8 hours. Stir well and serve.

Nutrition: Calories: 323 Fat: 12g Carbs: 6.2g Protein: 44.9g

Cilantro Lime Chicken

Preparation time: 10 minutes

Cooking time: 6 hours

Servings: 4 people

Ingredients:

- 6 chicken breasts, boneless
- 2 jalapeno peppers, chopped
- 1 1/4 oz taco seasoning
- 1/4 cup fresh cilantro, chopped
- 1 lime juice
- 24 oz salsa

Directions:

1. Add all fixings except chicken into the slow cooker and mix well. Add chicken into the slow cooker. Cover and cook on low within 6 hours. Shred chicken using a fork and serve.

Nutrition: Calories: 162 Fat: 5.9 g Carbs: 4.5 g Protein: 22.4 g

Garlic Chicken

Preparation time: 10 minutes

Cooking time: 6 hours

Servings: 4 people

Ingredients:

- 4 lbs. whole chicken
- 1 tsp dried oregano
- 1 tsp dried basil leaves
- 1 1/2 tsp dried thyme leaves
- 1 tbsp garlic, chopped
- 1 large onion, sliced
- 1/2 tsp pepper
- 1 tsp salt

Directions:

1. Place sliced onion into the slow cooker. Mix garlic, thyme, basil, oregano, pepper, and salt in a small bowl.

2. Rub garlic mixture all over chicken and place into the slow cooker. Cover and cook on low within 6 hours. Sliced and serve.

Nutrition:

Calories: 589

Fat: 22.5g

Carbs: 3.2g

Protein: 87.9g

Caribbean Jerk Chicken

Preparation time: 10 minutes

Cooking time: 6 hours

Servings: 4 people

Ingredients:

- 4 lbs. whole chicken
- 1/3 cup fresh lime juice
- 1/2 tsp cayenne pepper
- 1 tsp cinnamon
- 1 tbsp allspice
- 2 tsp kosher salt

Directions:

1. Mix allspice, cinnamon, cayenne pepper, and kosher salt in a small bowl. Rub spice mixture all over the chicken.

2. Place chicken into the slow cooker. Pour lime juice over the chicken. Cover and cook on low within 6 hours. Slice and serve.

Nutrition:

Calories: 437

Fat: 16.9g

Carbs: 1.1g

Protein: 65.7g

Balsamic Chicken

Preparation time: 10 minutes

Cooking time: 4 hours

Servings: 4 people

Ingredients:

- 2 1/2 lb. chicken thighs, skinless and boneless
- 1/4 cup fresh basil leaves, chopped
- 1/2 cup grape tomatoes, quartered
- 1 tsp garlic, chopped
- 1 1/4 cups balsamic vinaigrette dressing

Directions:

1. Spray slow cooker from inside with cooking spray. Place chicken into the slow cooker. Pour balsamic vinaigrette dressing and garlic over the chicken.

2. Cover and cook on low within 4 hours. Remove chicken from slow cooker and place on a serving dish. Top with basil and grape tomatoes. Serve and enjoy.

Nutrition:

Calories: 375

Fat: 15g

Carbs: 1.2g

Protein: 54.9g

Caesar Chicken

Preparation time: 15 minutes

Cooking time: 8 hours

Servings: 4 people

Ingredients:

- 4 chicken breasts, skinless and boneless
- 1/2 tsp dried parsley
- 1/4 cup fresh basil, chopped
- 3/4 cup creamy Caesar dressing
- 1/8 tsp black pepper
- 1/8 tsp salt

Directions:

1. Place chicken into the slow cooker. Add parsley, Caesar dressing, black pepper, and salt into the slow cooker. Cover and cook on low within 8 hours. Shred

the chicken using a fork. Garnish with basil and serve.

Nutrition:

Calories: 366

Fat: 21.9 g

Carbs: 4.6 g

Protein: 32.9 g

Cheesy Cheddar Chicken

Preparation time: 10 minutes

Cooking time: 6 hours

Servings: 4 people

Ingredients:

- 1 1/2 lbs. chicken tenderloins, boneless
- 1 cup cheddar cheese, shredded
- 1 oz ranch dressing
- 10 3/4 oz cream of chicken soup

Directions:

1. Place chicken into the slow cooker and sprinkle with ranch dressing. Pour chicken soup over the chicken. Cover and cook on low within 6 hours.
2. Sprinkle with shredded cheddar cheese and cover until cheese is melted. Serve and enjoy.

Nutrition: Calories: 349 Fat: 18.7 g Carbs: 4.4 g Protein: 38.8 g

Lemon Butter Chicken

Preparation time: 10 minutes

Cooking time: 4 hours

Servings: 4 people

Ingredients:

- 4 chicken breasts, skinless and boneless
- 2 lemon juice
- 1 oz Italian salad dressing mix
- 2 tbsp butter

Directions:

1. Place chicken into the slow cooker. Top with lemon juice and butter. Sprinkle Italian salad dressing over the chicken. Cover and cook on low within 4 hours. Serve and enjoy.

Nutrition:

Calories: 355 Fat: 17 g Carbs: 5 g Protein: 42.7 g

Tahini Chicken

Preparation time: 10 minutes

Cooking time: 8 hours

Servings: 4 people

Ingredients:

- 1 1/2 lbs. chicken thighs, skinless and boneless
- 1 tbsp shallot, grated
- 2 garlic cloves, minced
- 2 tbsp lemon juice
- 2 tsp lemon zest
- 3 tbsp water
- 3 tbsp olive oil
- 1/4 cup tahini
- 1/2 tsp salt

Directions:

1. Place chicken into the slow cooker. Pour remaining ingredients over the chicken. Cover and cook on low

within 8 hours. Shred the chicken using a fork and serve.

Nutrition:

Calories: 255

Fat: 15.6 g

Carbs: 2.2 g

Protein: 26g

Shredded Mexican Chicken

Preparation time: 10 minutes

Cooking time: 6 hours

Servings: 4 people

Ingredients:

- 4 lbs. chicken breasts, skinless and boneless
- 2 tbsp chili powder
- 1/4 tsp pepper
- 2 tsp coriander
- 2 tsp cumin
- 2 tsp garlic, minced
- 2 tbsp dried onion flakes
- 1 cup of water
- 15 oz can tomato sauce
- 1/4 tsp pepper
- 1/2 tsp salt

Directions:

1. Place chicken into the bottom of the slow cooker. Mix all remaining ingredients and pour over chicken. Cover and cook on low within 6 hours.
2. Remove chicken from slow cooker and shred the chicken using a fork, then return into the slow cooker and stir well. Serve and enjoy.

Nutrition:

Calories: 457

Fat: 17.4 g

Carbs: 5.4 g

Protein: 66.8 g

Parmesan Chicken Drumsticks

Preparation time: 10 minutes

Cooking time: 4 hours

Servings: 4 people

Ingredients:

- 5 lbs. chicken drumsticks
- 1 tbsp parsley, chopped
- 1/4 cup parmesan cheese, grated
- 1 tbsp garlic, minced
- 1 tbsp lemon juice
- 1/2 cup butter, melted
- 1 cup chicken broth
- 2 tsp onion powder
- 2 tsp garlic powder
- 2 tbsp olive oil
- 1/2 tsp pepper
- 1 tsp salt

Directions:

1. Coat chicken drumsticks with olive oil. In a small bowl, mix onion powder, garlic powder, pepper, and salt.
2. Sprinkle onion powder mixture over the chicken drumsticks. Place chicken drumsticks into the slow cooker.
3. Pour chicken broth into the slow cooker—cover and cook on high within 4 hours. Mix remaining ingredients and pour over chicken. Serve and enjoy.

Nutrition:

Calories: 465

Fat: 23.9 g

Carbs: 1.1 g

Protein: 56.7 g

Mediterranean Chicken

Preparation time: 10 minutes

Cooking time: 4 hours

Servings: 4 people

Ingredients:

- 4 chicken breasts, skinless and boneless
- 2 tbsp capers
- 1 small onion, chopped
- 1 tbsp garlic, minced
- 2 tbsp fresh lemon juice
- 1 cup roasted red peppers, chopped
- 1 cup olives
- 3 tsp Italian seasoning
- Pepper
- Salt

Directions:

1. Season chicken with pepper and salt. Cook the chicken in a pan over medium-high heat 2 minutes on each side until browned.
2. Transfer chicken into the slow cooker. Pour remaining ingredients over the chicken. Cover and cook on low within 4 hours. Serve and enjoy.

Nutrition:

Calories: 352

Fat: 15.7 g

Carbs: 8 g

Protein: 43.4 g

Lemon Garlic Chicken

Preparation time: 10 minutes

Cooking time: 5 hours

Servings: 4 people

Ingredients:

- 2 lbs. chicken breasts, skinless and boneless
- 3 tbsp fresh lemon juice
- 1/4 cup water
- 2 tbsp butter
- 1 tsp dried oregano
- 1 tbsp fresh parsley, chopped
- 1 tsp chicken bouillon granules
- 2 garlic cloves, minced
- 1/4 tsp black pepper
- 1/2 tsp salt

Directions:

1. Mix garlic, oregano, pepper, and salt in a small bowl. Rub garlic mixture all over chicken breasts.
2. Dissolve the butter in a large pan over medium heat—brown chicken in hot butter and place in the slow cooker's bottom.
3. Pour remaining ingredients over chicken. Cover and cook on low within 5 hours. Serve and enjoy.

Nutrition:

Calories: 326

Fat: 15.1 g

Carbs: 0.8 g

Protein: 44 g

Sweet & Smoky Pulled Chicken

Preparation time: 5 minutes

Cooking time: 7 hours & 5 minutes

Servings: 4 people

Ingredients:

- 1-pound pasture-raised chicken breasts, skinless
- 13 1/2 fluid ounce tomato passata, unsweetened
- 1 teaspoon garlic powder
- 1 teaspoon of sea salt
- 1 teaspoon ground black pepper
- ½ cup apple cider vinegar
- 3 tablespoon Swerve sweeteners
- 1/4 tsp cayenne pepper
- 1 tablespoon smoked paprika
- 3 tablespoons coconut aminos
- ½ cup avocado oil
- 1 cup sour cream for serving

Directions:

1. Put the chicken breast in your slow cooker. Whisk together remaining ingredients except for sour cream and pour over chicken.
2. Shut with lid and cook for 6 to 7 hours at low heat setting or 2 to 4 hours at high heat setting or until cooked. When done, transfer chicken to a cutting board and shred with two forks.
3. Transfer sauce in the slow cooker to a saucepan and simmer for 3 minutes or more.
4. Spoon this sauce over chicken, stir until chicken is coated with sauce. Add a little more oil, toss until combined, then top with sour cream and serve straightaway.

Nutrition:

Calories: 234

Fat: 12g

Protein: 27.5g

Carbs: 4g

Mexican Chicken Fajita Soup

Preparation time: 5 minutes

Cooking time: 6 hours

Servings: 4 people

Ingredients:

- 2 pasture-raised chicken breasts, skinless
- 2 tablespoons cashew butter
- 1 medium red bell pepper, diced
- 1/2 small white onion, diced
- 1 teaspoon minced garlic
- 10-ounce tomatoes & chilies
- 1 tablespoon taco seasoning
- 1 cup chicken broth
- 2/3 cup and 1 tablespoon cream cheese
- 1/2 cup heavy whipping cream
- 4 tablespoons sour cream for topping

Directions:

1. Put a large skillet pan on medium heat, add butter and when it melts, add pepper, onion, garlic, taco seasoning and cook for 3 minutes or until fragrant and onion are slightly tender.
2. Spoon this mixture in a 6-quart slow cooker, add chicken, tomato, chilies, and broth, and shut with lid. Plugin the slow cooker and cook chicken for 4 to 6 hours at a low heat setting or until chicken is tender.
3. When done, stir in cream cheese and heavy cream until creamy, then top with sour cream and serve.

Nutrition:

Calories: 476

Fat: 35.9g

Protein: 31.8g

Carbs: 10.8g

Creamy Tuscan Garlic Chicken

Preparation time: 15 minutes

Cooking time: 8 hours & 10 minutes

Servings: 4 people

Ingredients:

- 4 large pasture-raised chicken breast, each about 6 oz.
- 1/2 cup sun-dried tomatoes, chopped
- 2 cup spinach, chopped
- 3 teaspoons minced garlic
- 1 ½ teaspoon sea salt
- 1 teaspoon ground black pepper
- 1 tablespoon Italian seasoning
- 1 tablespoon avocado oil
- 1 cup heavy cream
- 1/3 cup chicken broth
- 3/4 cup grated parmesan cheese

Directions:

1. Put oil in your saucepan on medium heat, then put garlic and cook for 1 minute or until fragrant.
2. Whisk in cream and broth, bring the mixture to simmer, reduce heat to a low level, and simmer more for 10 minutes or until sauce thickens enough to coat the spoon's back.
3. In the meantime, place the chicken in a 6-quarts slow cooker. When the sauce is ready, stir in cheese until smooth, and then pour it over the chicken.
4. Cook within 6 to 8 hours at low heat setting or 3 to 4 hours at high heat setting or until cooked. When done, transfer chicken to a serving plate and set aside.
5. Add spinach to the sauce in the slow cooker and cook for 3 to 5 minutes or until spinach leaves wilt. Spoon sauce over chicken, then top with tomatoes and serve.

Nutrition: Calories: 531 Fat: 35g Protein: 45g Carbs: 9

Chicken Stew

Preparation time: 5 minutes

Cooking time: 2 hours & 10 minutes

Servings: 4 people

Ingredients:

- 28 oz. skinless pasture-raised chicken thighs, diced into 1-inch pieces
- ½ cup chopped white onion
- 1 cup fresh spinach
- 2 sticks of celery, diced
- 1 ½ teaspoon minced garlic
- 1 teaspoon salt
- ½ teaspoon ground black pepper
- ½ teaspoon dried rosemary
- ¼ teaspoon dried thyme
- ½ teaspoon dried oregano
- 2 cups chicken stock

- ½ cup heavy cream

Directions:

1. Place all the ingredients except for spinach and cream in a 6-quart slow cooker and shut with a lid. Cook for 4 hours at a low heat setting or 2 hours at a high heat setting or until cooked.
2. Then stir in spinach and cream and cook for 5 to 10 minutes at a high heat setting or until spinach leaves wilt. Serve straight away.

Nutrition:

Calories: 356

Fat: 24g

Protein: 31g

Carbs: 6g

Curried Chicken Tacos

Preparation time: 5 minutes

Cooking time: 8 hours

Servings: 4 people

Ingredients:

For Curried Chicken:

- 2 pounds skinless pasture-raised chicken breasts
- 15-ounce diced tomatoes
- 3 chilis de Arbol, chopped
- 1/2 of medium white onion, chopped
- 2 teaspoon grated ginger
- 2 teaspoons minced garlic
- 1 teaspoon salt
- 1 1/2 teaspoons ground turmeric
- 2 teaspoons ground cumin
- 1 tablespoon ground coriander
- 1/4 teaspoon cinnamon

- 1/4 teaspoon ground cardamom
- 2-star anise
- 1/2 cup chicken stock

For Avocado Cream:

- 1 large avocado, pitted
- 1/3 cup chopped cilantro
- 2 teaspoons onion powder
- 1/2 teaspoon salt
- 1 1/2 teaspoons red chili powder
- 5 tablespoons yogurt, high-fat
- 1 1/2 tablespoons lemon juice

For Taco:

- 1/2 of small red cabbage, sliced
- 8 large leaves of collard greens
- 1 large red pepper, sliced
- 2 cups sour cream

Directions:

1. Place all the ingredients, except for star anise, and stock in a 6-quart slow cooker and toss until just mixed. Then pour in chicken stock, add star anise, and shut with lid.
2. Cook within 7 to 8 hours at low heat setting or 4 to5 hours at high heat setting.
3. For the avocado cream, place the ingredients for avocado cream in a food processor and pulse for 1 to 2 minutes or until smooth; set aside until required.
4. Trim the tough stem from collard greens, rinse well, pat dry, and set aside until required. When chicken is cooked, shred with two forks and toss until coated with sauce.
5. Arrange collard greens in a clean working space, then top with chicken, cabbage, pepper, avocado cream, and sour cream in the end. Serve straight away.

Nutrition: Calories: 371.25 Fat: 19g Protein: 41g Carbs: 9g

Ranch Chicken

Preparation time: 5 minutes

Cooking time: 7 hours

Servings: 4 people

Ingredients:

- 2 pounds skinless pasture-raised chicken breast
- 3 tablespoons dried ranch dressing
- 3 tablespoons butter, chopped
- 4-ounce cream cheese, chopped

Directions:

1. Place chicken in a 6-quart slow cooker, scatter with butter and cream cheese, and sprinkle with ranch dressing.

2. Shut with lid, then plug in the slow cooker and cook for 4 hours at high heat setting or 5 to 7 hours at low heat setting or until cooked. Shred chicken with two forks and stirs until evenly coated and serve straightaway.

Nutrition:

Calories: 251.3

Fat: 12.9g

Protein: 33g

Carbs: 0.8g

Chicken and Sausage

Preparation time: 5 minutes

Cooking time: 6 hours

Servings: 4 people

Ingredients:

- 1 1/2-pound skinless pasture-raised chicken breasts
- 13-ounce smoked sausage
- 1 small white onion, diced
- 1 ½ teaspoon minced garlic
- 1/2 teaspoon salt
- 2 tablespoons mustard paste, sugar-free
- 1/2 cup white wine
- 8-ounce cream cheese softened
- 1 cup chicken stock
- Scallions for garnish

Directions:

1. Place chicken and sausage in a 6-quart slow cooker and top with onion. Whisk together garlic, salt, mustard, white wine, cream cheese, and chicken stock until smooth and pour this mixture all over the chicken.
2. Plugin the slow cooker, and cook for 5 to 6 hours or 4 hours at a high heat setting. Garnish with scallion and serve straight away.

Nutrition:

Calories: 561

Fat: 37.4g

Protein: 50.5g

Carbs: 5.6g

Crack Chicken

Preparation time: 5 minutes

Cooking time: 8 hours

Servings: 4 people

Ingredients:

- 2 pounds pasture-raised chicken breasts
- 8 slices of bacon, cooked and crumbled
- 2 tablespoons Ranch seasoning
- 1/2 cup chicken broth
- 8-ounce block of Cream cheese, cubed
- 1/2 cup shredded cheddar cheese

Directions:

1. Pour broth in a 6-quart slow cooker, stir in ranch dressing and then add chicken. Plugin the slow cooker, shut with lid, and cook for 4 hours at a high heat setting or 8 hours at low heat or until cooked.

2. When done, shred chicken with two forks, then add bacon, cream cheese, and cheddar cheese and stir until well combined.
3. Continue cooking for 5 to 10 minutes at a high heat setting or until cheese melts. Serve straight away.

Nutrition:

Calories: 331

Fat: 23g

Protein: 30g

Carbs: 1g

Cheesy Adobo Chicken

Preparation time: 5 minutes

Cooking time: 8 hours & 5 minutes

Servings: 4 people

Ingredients:

- 1-pound pasture-raised chicken breasts, skin on
- 2 tablespoons adobo sauce
- 1/2 cup salsa, sugar-free

For Cheese Sauce:

- 1 tablespoon arrowroot powder
- 1 tablespoon unsalted butter
- 1/2 cup coconut milk, unsweetened and full-fat
- 6 tablespoons grated cheddar cheese
- 6 tablespoons grated Monterey jack cheese

Directions:

1. Place adobo sauce and salsa in a 6-quart slow cooker, whisk together until combined, and then add chicken.

2. Plugin the slow cooker, shut with lid and cook for 6 to 8 hours at low heat setting or 3 to 4 hours at high heat setting or until cooked. Shred chicken with two forks and tosses until mixed with the sauce.

3. Prepare cheese sauce and for this, place a medium saucepan over medium-high heat, add butter and when it melts, whisk in arrowroot powder and simmer for 1 minute.

4. Then slowly whisk in milk until smooth and cook for 4 minutes or until sauce thickens slightly. Remove saucepan from heat, add cheese and stir well until cheese melts and the smooth sauce comes together. Pour cheese over chicken and serve.

Nutrition: Calories: 313 Fat: 21g Protein: 26g Carbs: 5g

Green Beans & Chicken Thighs

Preparation time: 5 minutes

Cooking time: 8 hours

Servings: 4 people

Ingredients:

- 4 skin-on pasture-raised chicken thighs
- 1-pound green beans, trimmed
- 2 large tomatoes, diced
- 1 medium white onion, peeled and diced
- 1 teaspoon minced garlic
- 2 teaspoons salt and more for seasoning chicken
- 1 teaspoon ground black pepper and more for seasoning chicken
- 1/4 cup fresh chopped dill
- 6 tablespoons avocado oil, divided
- 1 lemon, juiced
- 1 cup chicken broth

- 1 cup sour cream

Directions:

1. Place green beans in a 6-quarts slow cooker, add remaining ingredients except for 3 tablespoons oil, chicken, and sour cream and stir until mixed.
2. Plugin slow cooker, top green beans with chicken, drizzle with oil, season with salt and black pepper, and shut with lid.
3. Cook for 8 hours at a low heat setting or 4 hours at a high heat setting or until chicken is cooked through. Serve with sour cream.

Nutrition:

Calories: 622

Fat: 46.3g

Protein: 35.7g

Carbs: 15.5g

Pizza Chicken

Preparation time: 5 minutes

Cooking time: 3 hours & 30 minutes

Servings: 4 people

Ingredients:

- 4 skinless pasture-raised chicken breasts
- 20 slices of pepperoni
- 1 ½ teaspoon salt
- 1 teaspoon ground black pepper
- 2 cups marinara sauce, sugar-free
- 1 cup grated parmesan cheese

Directions:

1. Spread marinara sauce into a 6-quart slow cooker, then add chicken and season with salt and black

pepper. Plugin the slow cooker, top chicken with pepperoni slices, and shut with lid.

2. Cook chicken for 3 hours at a low heat setting, then add cheese and continue cooking for 15 to 30 minutes. Serve straight away.

Nutrition:

Calories: 418

Fat: 20g

Protein: 49g

Carbs: 10.5g

Chicken with Bacon Gravy

Preparation time: 5 minutes

Cooking time: 3 hours & 30 minutes

Servings: 4 people

Ingredients:

- 1 ½ pound skinless pasture-raised chicken breasts
- 6 slices of bacon, cooked and crumbled
- 1 teaspoon minced garlic
- ¼ teaspoon ground black pepper
- 1 teaspoon dried thyme
- 3 ½ tablespoons dried chicken gravy mix
- 4 tablespoons oil
- 1¼ cup of water
- 1 cup heavy cream

Directions:

1. Place chicken in a 4-quart slow cooker, add bacon and sprinkle with garlic, black pepper, and garlic, and drizzle with oil.
2. Whisk together water and chicken gravy mix until smooth, and then pour this mixture over the chicken.
3. Plugin the slow cooker, shut with lid, and cook for 3 ½ hours at a high heat setting or until chicken is cooked.
4. When done, add cream, then shred chicken with 2 forks and stir until well combined. Serve straight away.

Nutrition:

Calories: 551

Fat: 38g

Protein: 51g

Carbs: 1.3g

Chicken Lo Mein

Preparation time: 15 minutes

Cooking time: 4 hours & 10 minutes

Servings: 4 people

Ingredients:

- 1 1/2 pounds boneless pasture-raised chicken thighs, sliced
- 12 oz. kelp noodles
- 1 bunch bok choy, sliced
- 1 teaspoon minced garlic
- 1 teaspoon grated ginger
- 1 ½ teaspoon salt
- ¾ teaspoon ground black pepper

For Chicken Marinade:

- 1/2 teaspoon minced garlic
- 1 tablespoon coconut aminos
- 1/2 teaspoon avocado oil

For Sauce:

- 1/2 teaspoon xanthan gum
- 1 tablespoon swerve sweetener
- 1 teaspoon red pepper chili flakes
- 1/4 cup coconut aminos
- 2 teaspoon sesame oil
- 1 tablespoon apple cider vinegar
- 3/4 cup chicken broth

Directions:

1. Place all the ingredients for the marinade in a large bowl, whisk until combined, then add chicken, toss until well coated, and let marinate in the refrigerator for 30 minutes.
2. Then grease a 6-quart slow cooker with oil, add marinated chicken, and shut with lid. Cook within 2 hours at a low heat setting or for 1 hour at high heat.
3. Move the cooked chicken to a serving plate and add cabbage, ginger, garlic to the slow cooker, and top with chicken.

4. Whisk the sauce ingredients in a bowl, pour all over the chicken, and shut with lid—Cook for 1 hour to 2 hours on low or 30 minutes to 1 hour on high.
5. In the meantime, rinse kelp noodles and soak them in water. When cooking time is up, add kelp noodles to the slow cooker and stir with tongs until evenly coated with sauce.
6. Stir in xanthan gum and cook for 10 to 15 minutes on high. Serve straight away.

Nutrition:

Calories: 198

Fat: 10.1g

Protein: 24.5g

Carbs: 3.1g

Chicken Bacon Chowder

Preparation time: 5 minutes

Cooking time: 9 hours & 5 minutes

Servings: 4 people

Ingredients:

- 1-pound pasture-raised chicken breast, skinless
- 1-pound bacon
- 6-ounce Cremini mushrooms
- 2 celery, diced
- 1 medium white onion, peeled and diced
- 2 teaspoons minced garlic
- 1 teaspoon garlic powder
- 1 teaspoon salt
- 1 teaspoon ground black pepper
- 1 teaspoon dried thyme
- 2 tablespoons avocado oil
- 2 tablespoons unsalted butter

- 2 cups chicken stock
- 8-ounce cream cheese, cubed
- 1 cup heavy cream

Directions:

1. Plug in a 6-quart slow cooker and let preheat at a low heat setting. Then add mushrooms, celery, onion, garlic, salt, black pepper, butter, and 1 cup stock and stir until mixed.
2. Shut with lid and cook for 1 hour at a low heat setting. Place a large skillet pan over medium-high heat, add oil and when hot, add oil and when hot, put the chicken and cook within 5 minutes or until seared on all sides.
3. Transfer seared chicken to a plate, deglaze the pan with remaining stock and stir well to remove browned bits stuck on the pan's bottom, and then add to slow cooker when vegetables are cooked.
4. Add remaining ingredients to cooked vegetables, stir well until cream cheese is mixed. Cut chicken into

cubes, add to slow cooker along with bacon, and stir until mixed.

5. Shut with lid and cook for 6 to 8 hours at a low heat setting or until cooked. Serve.

Nutrition:

Calories: 879.3

Fat: 66.4g

Protein: 59.3g

Carbs: 11g

Sesame Ginger Chicken

Preparation time: 5 minutes

Cooking time: 6 hours

Servings: 4 people

Ingredients:

- 1 ½ pound skinless pasture-raised chicken breasts
- 2 tablespoons chopped red bell pepper
- ¼ cup minced onion
- 1 teaspoon minced garlic
- ½ tablespoon grated fresh ginger
- ½ teaspoon crushed red pepper flakes
- 1 tablespoon swerve sweetener
- 2 tablespoons coconut aminos
- 3 tablespoons sesame seed oil
- ½ cup tomato puree
- 1/3 cup peach jam, sugar-free
- 1/3 cup chicken broth

- 2 teaspoons sesame seeds

Directions:

1. Place all the fixings in a 6-quart slow cooker, except for sesame seeds, chicken, and pepper, and stir until mixed.
2. Add chicken, turn to coat chicken with sauce and then top with red bell pepper. Plugin the slow cooker, shut with lid, and cook for 6 hours at low heat setting or 4 hours at high heat setting. Garnish with sesame seeds and serve.

Nutrition:

Calories: 180

Fat: 12.8g

Protein: 37.8g

Carbs: 2g

Coco Loco Chicken Curry

Preparation time: 15 minutes

Cooking time: 5 hours

Servings: 4 people

Ingredients:

- 6 boneless chicken thighs
- 13½ oz. coconut milk
- 1 tbsp. curry powder
- 2 tbsps. coconut oil
- 1 tbsp. minced garlic
- 1 chopped jalapeno
- sea salt
- 2 tsp. almond flour
- 1 cup lime juice
- 20 fresh basil leaves

Directions:

1. Put the chicken in the slow cooker and pour the milk all over it. Cook the chicken on high for 4 hours.
2. Meanwhile, in a saucepan over medium-high heat, add in the coconut oil. Once it melts, toss in the garlic and jalapeno peppers. Sauté it for 2-3 minutes.
3. Add the curry powder, salt, and almond flour, then simmer for 2 minutes. Pour the curry mixture over the chicken.
4. Let it simmer for 45-60 minutes. Once cooked, add the basil and lime juice. You may opt to shred the chicken before serving.

Nutrition:

Calories: 351

Fat: 36.5g

Carbs: 6.0g

Protein: 17.1g

Ranch Chicken with Broccoli

Preparation time: 10 minutes

Cooking time: 5 hours

Servings: 4 people

Ingredients:

Homemade ranch seasoning:

- ½ tsp garlic powder
- 1½ tsp Dill, dry
- 1 tbsp dried parsley
- 2 tsp dried chives
- ½ tsp. paprika
- sea salt
- black pepper

Chicken:

- 3 boneless chicken breasts
- 12 slices bacon
- 1 tbsp homemade seasoning

- 1½ tsp steak seasoning
- 6 cups broccoli florets
- ½ cup mayonnaise
- 3 tbsps. red wine vinegar
- ¼ tsp. sea salt
- Hot sauce

Directions:

1. Mix the ranch seasoning ingredients in a bowl. Transfer it to a small jar with a tight cap. Put the chicken in your slow cooker. Season it with ranch and steak seasonings. Cook it on low for 4 hours.
2. Toss the broccoli into the pot. Let it cook for another 30-60 minutes. Transfer chicken to a bowl once cooked, and shred it using 2 forks. Mix in the broccoli, mayo, vinegar, and hot sauce.

Nutrition: Calories: 239 Fat: 21.3g Carbs: 7.8g Protein: 18.7g

Garlic Parmesan Chicken Wings

Preparation time: 10 minutes

Cooking time: 2 hours & 50 minutes

Servings: 2 people

Ingredients:

- 8 tbsps. butter
- 2 minced garlic cloves
- 1 tbsp. Italian seasoning, dried
- ¼ cup parmesan cheese, grated
- Sea salt
- Black pepper
- 1 lb. chicken wings

Directions:

1. Set slow cooker to high. Line an aluminum foil on the baking sheet. Put the butter, garlic, Italian seasoning, and ¼ cup of parmesan cheese in the slow cooker,

and season with pink salt and pepper. Dissolve the butter, and stir the ingredients until well mixed.

2. Add the chicken wings and stir until coated with the butter mixture. Cook for 2 hours and 45 minutes while the slow cooker is covered.

3. Preheat the broiler. Move the wings on your prepared baking sheet, sprinkle the remaining ½ cup of Parmesan cheese over the wings, and cook under the broiler until crispy, about 5 minutes. Serve hot.

Nutrition:

Calories: 738

Fat: 66g

Carbs: 4g

Protein: 39g

Luau Chicken

Preparation time: 15 minutes

Cooking time: 6 hours

Servings: 4 people

Ingredients:

- 6 bacon strips
- 6 boneless chicken thighs
- Salt
- Pepper
- ½ cup red onion
- 1 cup sliced pineapple

Directions:

1. Place half of the bacon strips in a skillet over medium flame and cook until crispy. Drain and set aside on a paper towel.

2. Season the chicken with salt and pepper. Place inside the slow cooker and top with half of the uncooked bacon. Top with onions and pineapples.
3. Cook within 6 hours or until the chicken is very tender. Top with crumbled crispy bacon before serving.

Nutrition:

Calories: 375

Carbs: 8g

Protein: 39g

Fat: 17g

Southwest Chicken

Preparation time: 10 minutes

Cooking time: 5 hours

Servings: 4 people

Ingredients:

- 1 chopped zucchini
- 1 jar sugar-free salsa
- 4 boneless chicken breasts
- 1 cubed red bell pepper
- Salt
- Pepper

Directions:

1. Place half of the zucchini at the bottom of the slow cooker. Pour over half of the salsa. Then arrange the chicken breasts and bell peppers on top.

2. Continue to layer until all ingredients are inside the slow cooker—season with salt and pepper to taste. Cook within 5 hours on low or until chicken is tender.
3. Give a good stir to mix everything. Serve with cilantro, sour cream, or cheese.

Nutrition:

Calories: 234

Carbs: 13g

Protein: 24g

Fat: 10g

Carolina-Style Vinegar Chicken

Preparation time: 10 minutes

Cooking time: 6 hours

Servings: 4 people

Ingredients:

- 1 cup white vinegar
- ¼ cup yacon syrup
- 1 tbsp. low sodium chicken stock
- 1½ lb. boneless chicken breast
- Salt
- pepper

Directions:

1. Use a small bowl, mix the white vinegar, yacon syrup, and chicken stock. Place the chicken breasts skin-side up inside the slow cooker. Pour over the mixture.

2. Season with salt and pepper to taste. Cook for 6 hours on low or until the chicken is tender. Shred the chicken meat apart using a fork. Serve on top of lettuce leaves.

Nutrition:

Calories: 188

Carbs: 3g

Protein: 26g

Fat: 12g

Chicken Cacciatore with Zoodles

Preparation time: 15 minutes

Cooking time: 6-7 hours & 8 minutes

Servings: 4 people

Ingredients:

- 2 lbs. minced chicken
- 1 cup chicken stock
- 1 cup chopped tomatoes
- 2 tbsps. olive oil
- ½ cup sliced onions
- 3 minced garlic cloves
- 1 tsp. oregano, dry
- 1 tsp. thyme, dry
- 1 tsp. parsley, dry
- salt
- Parmesan cheese

For zoodles:

- 1 washed and trimmed zucchini
- 2 tsp coconut oil

Directions:

1. Using a spiralizer, create zucchini noodles (zoodles). Heat coconut oil in a non-stick pan. Place the zoodles into the pan. Cook briefly for 3–5 minutes, depending on how tender you prefer the zoodles.
2. Heat the oil in the slow cooker on high. Put the onions and cook until they are golden brown. Add the chicken mince and garlic and cook for another 3 minutes.
3. Mix the remaining fixings in a large mixing bowl and add them to the chicken. Cook on low for about 6–7 hours. Serve hot over zoodles, with some grated Parmesan cheese if desired.

Nutrition: Calories: 347 Fat: 17g Carbs: 6g Protein: 28g

Bok Choy Chicken

Preparation time: 15 minutes

Cooking time: 6 hours & 30 minutes

Servings: 4 people

Ingredients:

- 6 lbs. cubed boneless chicken
- 8 oz. sliced bok choy
- 2 chopped green onions
- 2 tbsps. olive oil
- 1 tbsp. chopped ginger
- 2 minced garlic cloves
- 1 tbsp. soy sauce
- black pepper
- 2 tsp. paprika
- salt
- ½ cup of water

Directions:

1. Combine the chicken, onion, oil, ginger, garlic, soy sauce, black pepper, paprika, salt, and water in a slow cooker. Cook on high for 6 hours. Add the bok choy and cook for extra 30 minutes. Serve hot.

Nutrition:

Calories: 278

Fat: 18g

Carbs: 5g

Protein: 30g

Chicken Tikka Masala

Preparation time: 15 minutes

Cooking time: 6 hours

Servings: 4 people

Ingredients:

- 3 lbs. cubed chicken
- 1 cup diced tomatoes
- 2 tbsp olive oil
- 1 chopped onion
- 3 minced garlic cloves
- 1 tsp ground ginger
- 3 tbsp tomato paste
- 2 tsp smoked paprika
- 1 tsp cumin powder
- ¼ cup garam masala
- 1 cup heavy cream
- 1 cup of coconut milk

- 1 tsp salt
- Fresh coriander

Directions:

1. Add the oil, chicken, and all the dry spices to the slow cooker. Add the diced tomatoes, onion, ginger, garlic, tomato paste, salt, and coconut milk. Mix thoroughly.
2. Cook for 6 hours on low. Add in the heavy cream and mix. Garnish with some fresh coriander and cream.

Nutrition:

Calories: 219

Fat: 20g

Carbs: 5g

Protein: 41g

Chili Lime Chicken Wings

Preparation time: 15 minutes

Cooking time: 6 hours & 15 minutes

Servings: 4 people

Ingredients:

- 2 lbs. chicken wings
- ¼ cup fresh lime juice
- 4 minced garlic cloves
- 1 tbsp. chopped ginger
- 1 tbsp. chili sauce
- ¼ cup coconut aminos
- 1 tbsp. fish sauce
- ¼ cup coconut oil
- 1 tsp. oregano, dry
- black pepper
- salt
- Sliced lemon

Directions:

1. Preheat the slow cooker on high. Mix all the fixings until well combined in a large bowl. Transfer into the slow cooker. Cook for 6 hours on high.
2. Preheat the oven to 350°F. Transfer the wings onto a parchment-lined baking tray. Bake for 15 minutes until nicely golden brown. Serve hot with some lemon slices.

Nutrition:

Calories: 176

Fat: 9g

Carbs: 4g

Protein: 30g

Garlic Chicken & Mushroom Chowder

Preparation time: 15 minutes

Cooking time: 9 hours

Servings: 4 people

Ingredients:

- 6 oz. sliced Cremini mushrooms
- 1 lb. chicken breasts
- 4 minced garlic cloves
- 1 chopped shallot
- 1 sliced leek
- 2 diced celery ribs
- 1 sliced sweet onion
- 4 tbsps. Butter
- 2 cups chicken stock
- 8 oz. cream cheese

- 1 cup heavy cream
- 1 lb. crumbled bacon
- sea salt
- black pepper
- 1 tsp. garlic powder
- 1 tsp. thyme, dry

Directions:

1. Combine the leek, garlic, shallots, celery, onions, mushrooms, 1 cup chicken stock, salt, pepper, and 2 tablespoon butter in a slow cooker and cook covered for 1 hour on low.
2. Melt the remaining butter in a skillet and sear the chicken breasts in it. Chop into cubes. Remove the chicken and deglaze the skillet using the chicken stock.

3. Add the chicken along with the chicken stock to the slow cooker. Stir in the rest of the ingredients. Cook covered for 6-8 hours on low.

Nutrition:

Calories: 355

Fat: 28g

Carbs: 6.4g

Protein: 21 g

Saucy Duck

Preparation time: 10 minutes

Cooking time: 6 hours

Servings: 4 people

Ingredients:

- 1 duck, cut into small chunks
- 4 garlic cloves, minced
- 4 tablespoons of swerves
- 2 green onions, roughly diced
- 4 tablespoon of soy sauce
- 4 tablespoon of sherry wine
- 1/4 cup of water
- 1-inch ginger root, sliced
- A pinch salt
- black pepper to taste

Directions:

1. Put all the fixings into the slow cooker and mix them well. Cover it and cook for 6 hours on low. Garnish as desired. Serve warm.

Nutrition:

Calories: 338

Fat: 3.8g

Carbs: 8.3g

Protein: 15.4g

www.ingramcontent.com/pod-product-compliance
Lightning Source LLC
Chambersburg PA
CBHW071111030426
42336CB00013BA/2043